CONTENTS

Fitness Foundry

PRESENTS....

BREAK OUT OF...
BREAKING EVEN!

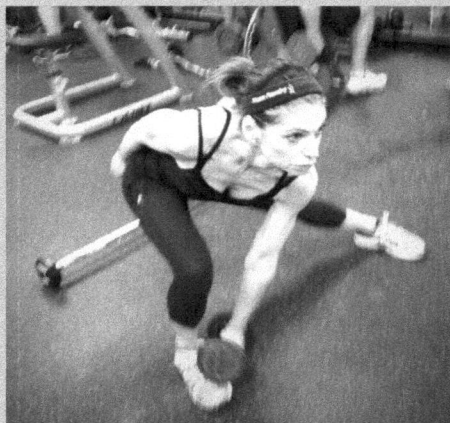

3-STEP METHOD FOR PROVEN LONG-TERM WEIGHT LOSS

DESIGNED FOR YOUR LIFESTYLE AND GOALS!

BY JULIO A. SALADO NSCA-CPT

ISBN: 978-0-9993203-0-3

Chapter 1

INTRODUCTION

Congratulations on deciding to achieve your weight loss goal!

Let's get to the point: Would you like to learn how to break out of *"breaking even"*?

"Breaking even" is when you invest time in exercising and eating healthy but do not see results, especially long term results.

A prime example of *"breaking even"* would be exercising five days a week and overindulging on the weekend. The caloric expenditure from your weekly exercise was offset by all extra calories you consumed, perhaps without even noticing.

A second example is eating healthfully, complying with a diet, and exercising as often as possible but having rollercoaster weight loss and gains.

By using the simple tools in this book, you will be empowered and able to make better decisions to stay on track to reach your goals.

Real people, real results:

Maggie, Age 38, Female, Ht 5' 9", Sedentary Job, Full-Time Professional, Vegetarian

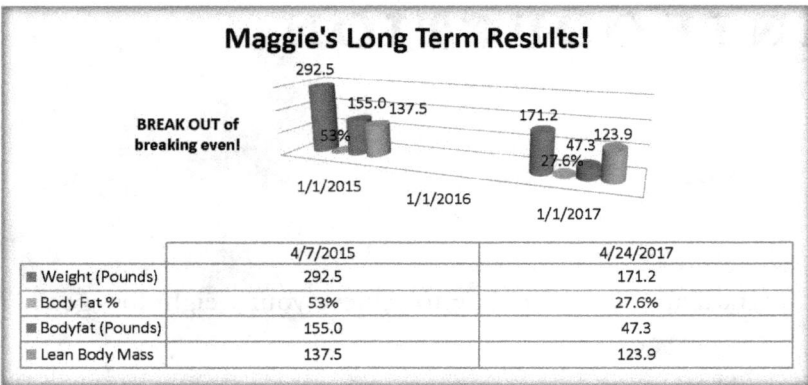

Maggie's Long Term Results!

	4/7/2015	4/24/2017
■ Weight (Pounds)	292.5	171.2
■ Body Fat %	53%	27.6%
■ Bodyfat (Pounds)	155.0	47.3
■ Lean Body Mass	137.5	123.9

Why is this book different from other weight loss programs?

I promote a three-step method that develops skills and self awareness for long-term weight loss management. The program is designed to be sustainable, flexible, and customized to fit your lifestyle and goals.

It's important to note that the emphasis this book is **weight loss management,** rather than sports performance.

Following this program you will learn how best to eat and exercise to promote fat loss.

Maggie's 107.7lbs Fat loss!

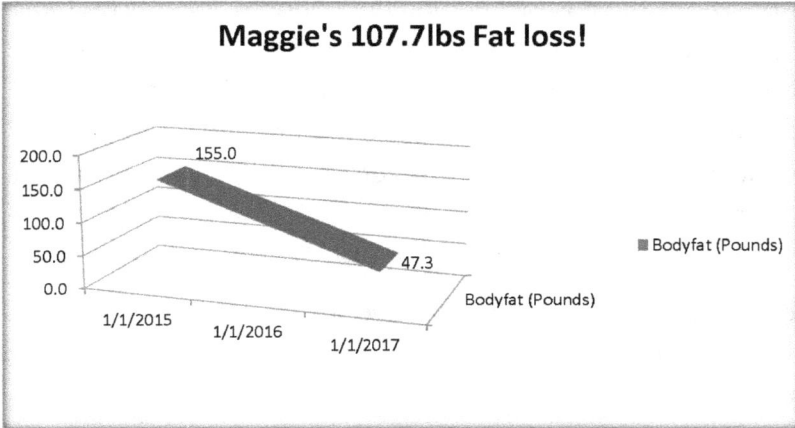

Why do people fail when working toward long-term weight loss?

"Training without a purpose"

People fail to reach their goals because they are breaking even and not optimizing their time. They are uneducated on their needed daily/weekly caloric deficit and are *"training without a purpose*"*

"Training with a purpose" is exercising along with implementing a nutrition plan that is designed for a specific, measureable, realistic goal. Our **"training purpose"** is weight loss.

"Prior to my using the A.I.M Method, I would say I was dedicated to working out with some frequency (three to five times per week), but it wasn't getting me where I wanted to be. I was just maintaining my weight. I am an avid bike rider, did a couple of barre classes a week, and muddled through my own weight workouts. But it had no focus, and I just thought given my frequency with working out, I couldn't lose any weight because I had hit a fitness plateau." —Jane

Your weight loss goal will no longer be solely dependent on one diet, running sprints, or a gimmicky abdominal crunch tool for losing weight.

What is the A.I.M. Method?

A program that teaches you about your innate potential and helps you optimize your results.

Assess your goals and use science-based tools to personalize and create a realistic and measurable program.

Commit: Take responsibility for your weight loss through a series of small consistent actions with a timeline.

Initiate the customized nutrition and exercise prescription with a purpose.

Connect: Engage your mind and body in a balanced three-step approach to nutrition, cardio, and strength training for weight loss.

Motivation will be gained from learning how to overcome your own challenges and avoid common setbacks.

Change: Use your motivation and understanding of key weight management concepts to achieve your personal goals.

You will also get practical tips, fitness facts, and support to maximize the tools and keep you on the road to success.

"Then came the incorporation of nutrition into the fitness picture. I wouldn't say I was a bad eater, but when I had a caloric goal, put that side by side with my activities, and understood that if I wanted to lose weight there were parameters I had to work within, it all started to click. It's not about starving myself. It's about being smarter about what I was eating, from portion sizes to more protein and tracking my exercise and my food intake." — Jane Lost 10 pounds in 12 weeks.

The A.I.M method has 3 facets that include a personalized approach to nutrition, cardio programming and strength training. It is designed to achieve long term goal.

Personalized for your lifestyle and Result Driven:

A.I.M. Method is NOT a diet nor is it a linear weight loss process. Any setbacks will become learning experiences on how to overcome challenges whether you have sugar cravings, can't find the time to work out, or feel unsure how to begin. *Let the A.I.M. Method navigate you through your weight loss journey and become the compass to help you reach your goal.*

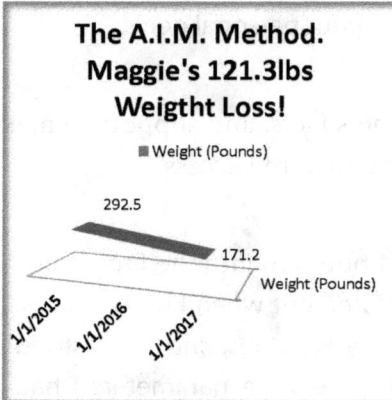

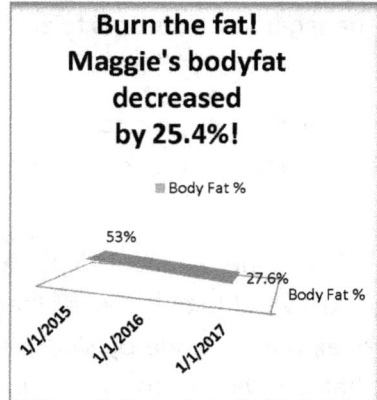

**The A.I.M. Method.
Maggie's 121.3lbs
Weigtht Loss!**

■ Weight (Pounds)

292.5

171.2

Weight (Pounds)

1/1/2015   1/1/2016   1/1/2017

**Burn the fat!
Maggie's bodyfat
decreased
by 25.4%!**

■ Body Fat %

53%

27.6%

Body Fat %

1/1/2015   1/1/2016   1/1/2017

"I believe using the A.I.M. Method designed by Julio Salado has educated me to make life changes that I will carry forward."
—Jane

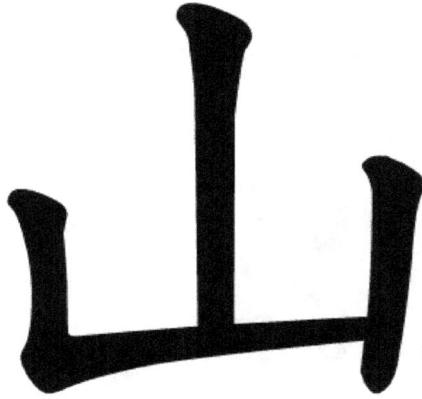

"Habit is the intersection of knowledge (what to do), skill (how to do), and desire (want to do)."
— Stephen R. Covey

Chapter 2

HEALTHY WEIGHT LOSS EXPECTATIONS AND COMMON EXCUSES

First things first! Let's start with the simple math on losing weight.

1 pound of fat = 3500 calories (approximate)

> Regardless of the brand, whether it's a points system, a high-protein diet, or a 12-week workout program all will have the same principle in common:
>
> Caloric deficit! Caloric deficit! Caloric deficit!

The distinction between a pound of fat and muscle is the density and volume. An easy way to understand the difference is the following: five pounds of fat takes up as much volume as three grapefruits, and five pounds of muscle takes up as much volume as three tangerines.

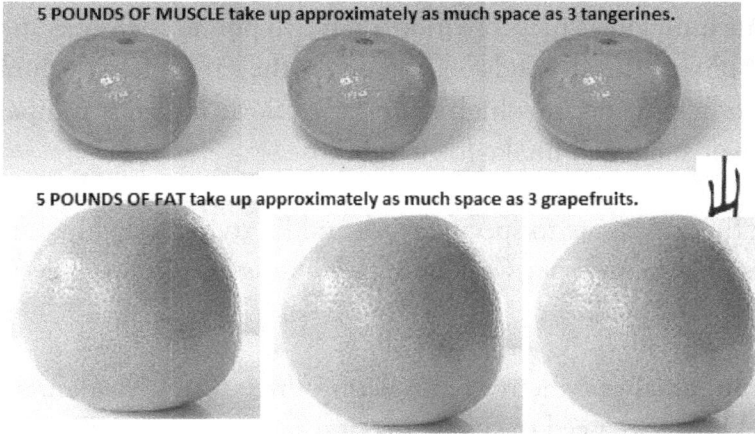

5 POUNDS OF MUSCLE take up approximately as much space as 3 tangerines.

5 POUNDS OF FAT take up approximately as much space as 3 grapefruits.

Your body requires more calories to sustain muscle than fat. Therefore, appropriate strength training exercises are an important component of this program.

A very common side effect of "diet only" weight loss is the loss of lean muscle mass. Our goal is to preserve and increase lean muscle in order to keep your metabolism running at its peak.

Cardio **does not** assist in increasing metabolism!

We will minimize muscle loss by avoiding an extreme caloric deficit (unsustainable diets), an emphasis on realistic caloric deficit via nutrition, rest, and combining appropriate resistance exercise and cardio.

Most people can expect to lose one to two pounds per week. Your weekly results will be contingent on meeting your personalized total weekly caloric deficit.

Some individuals may lose more than two pounds per week in the first phase. This depends on how active they are before beginning the program and how high their daily caloric intake is compared to their suggested intake for weight loss.

In other cases due to specific work and lifestyles, individuals may lose a half pound per week and with consistency can achieve any weight loss goal.

If you are already active (completing three to five workouts per week) then we need to channel your discipline and energy toward a program specifically designed for fat loss.

We will achieve the minimum weekly caloric deficit of 3500 calories through the following:

Nutrition: We will create a reasonable caloric deficit based on your Basal Metabolic Rate (BMR), lifestyle, and goal.

Cardiovascular exercises: We will identify which equipment will achieve the necessary caloric expenditure and time efficiency.

Resistance training: We will identify what exercises will achieve the necessary caloric expenditure and time efficiency plus burn calories up to 48 hours post workout.

Matt, Age 38, Ht 5' 10", Male, Sedentary Job, Full-Time Professional, Travels for Work, Two Young Kids.

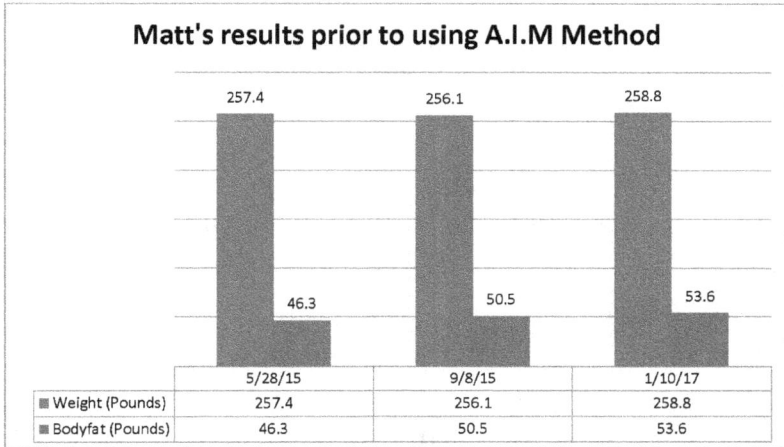

Matt's results prior to using A.I.M Method

	5/28/15	9/8/15	1/10/17
Weight (Pounds)	257.4	256.1	258.8
Bodyfat (Pounds)	46.3	50.5	53.6

Prior to 1/10/2017 he was "breaking even" and not losing weight. He stayed for two years at the same weight!

Matt's results AFTER using A.I.M Method.
Lost 27.8lbs in 4 Months!

	1/10/17	1/31/17	2/7/17	2/28/17	3/7/17	3/21/17	4/4/17	4/11/17	4/18/17	4/25/17
Weight	258.8	247.7	248	242.1	240.1	239.2	236.9	232.7	236	231.7

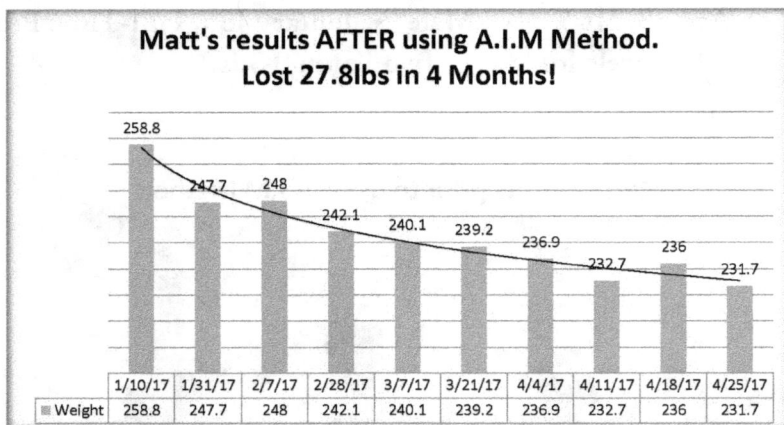

Your success lies in patience, consistency, and outside support. There is a learning curve with this system, but once you have mastered the basics, amazing results are possible!

The A.I.M. Method is flexible, so when life events happen the tools are still there!

Week after week, you will become better at hitting your daily goals and identifying which of the three steps are the most challenging.

Small changes can lead to BIG results. It may be an additional 30 minutes of cardio, eliminating a sports drink, or changing from doing only biceps curls to squats to overhead presses.

You will no longer lose or gain weight without understanding why and learning to overcome it!

What are the most common excuses for not achieving a weight loss goal?

Too overweight
Love Carbs
Lactose intolerant
Too Old
???

I eat out all the time
Travel for work
I have kids and too many temptations
Too much work, no time to workout
I am a picky eater
I have tried all diets and none work

The A.I.M. method is designed to be realistic and sustainable for every individual's lifestyle and goals.

山

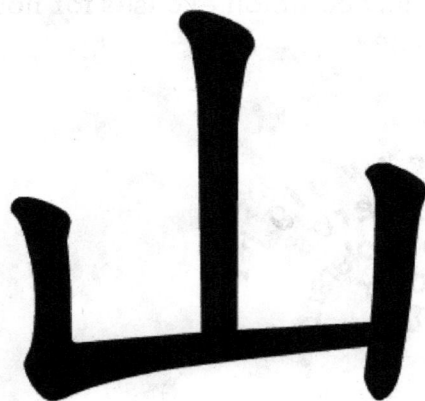

"If you fail to plan,
you are planning to fail!"
— BENJAMIN FRANKLIN

Chapter 3

ASSESS: WHEN WILL YOU HIT YOUR GOAL?

One of my goals in writing this book is to give you practical information that can be used today!

I will give simple insights into the science of weight loss without delving into unnecessary academic terms.

I encourage you to research the terms and methods used in this book to deepen your own understanding.

After you hit your short-term weight loss goal, you can then focus on body sculpting, which will lead to you to the science of nutrition macros and other modes of fitness.

> Female, Three Kids, Full-Time Job, Exercises 2x Per Week—Lost 10 pounds at a half pound per week
>
> "Thank you so much for the encouragement, for the plan, and for positively pushing me each week. Although it doesn't seem like much weight, it was a 10-pound start on weight that I couldn't manage to lose over years! I really thought this goal wasn't achievable with my work/family situation. Really can't thank you enough!" —Meghan, April 2017

Now let's get the data to help you "BREAK OUT of breaking even"!

You can also visit www.fitnessfoundry.net and use my online sheet to gather the data.

What you need for this section:

1. Calculator

2. Pen and paper

3. Scale and/or tape measurement, body fat calipers, body fat analyzer

4. Open-mindedness and honesty

Questionnaire A

Always get medical clearance prior to participating in any fitness or nutritional program.

BREAK OUT of Breaking Even Questionnaire:

Name:	Date:
Age:	Weight: Body fat % if available:
Gender:	Height: Height in Centimeters (inches x 2.54)

Q1. How many days per week can you REALISTICALLY work out?
Q2. What is the duration of your workout?
Q3. Short-term weight loss goal (1–3 months)?
Q4. Long-term weight loss goal (1 year +)?
Q5. Do you have access to a gym? If yes, what is your favorite cardio equipment and why?

Q6. If you have access to a gym do you only take group exercises classes? If no, what other exercises do you do on your own?

Q7. Have you ever tracked your calories and/or activities? If so, did you use an app or pen and paper?

Q7A. Do you know your current daily caloric intake? If so, please note.

Q8. When was the last time you felt your best?

Q9. What do you attribute your past success to?

Q10. Are you ready to commit to a new fitter, healthier, and leaner YOU? Please sign and date.

Sheet available online at www.fitnessfoundry.net

Let's plug in your answers to the formulas to create your personalized **A.I.M. Method** to help you hit your weight loss goal!

It's important to know the difference between your short- and long-term goals.

This will help to manage your expectations.

Step 1: How many calories do you need to burn to hit your SHORT-term goal?

To better assist you in understanding the steps, I will use a case study to demonstrate the process.

Case Study: Candie

- Age 35, Ht 5' 6" or 167.6 cm, Current Weight 200 Pounds or 90 Kilos, Body Fat 30% (optional if known)

- Exercises one to two times per week, leads a sedentary lifestyle

- Short-term weight loss goal: 190 pounds (10-pound loss)

- Long-term weight loss goal: 180 pounds (20-pound loss)

Here is the formula to learn how many calories of fat you need to scorch for the SHORT-term goal!

Exercise A1:

1. Formula: Current weight minus **short** term weight goal = Pounds of fat you need to BURN 2. Pounds of fat x 3,500 = Amount of calories you need to burn to hit short-term goal	
Candie 1. 200–190 = **10 pounds** 2. 10 x 3500 = 35,000 calories	**Candie needs to burn 35,000 calories over a period of time to lose 10 pounds.**
Enter your data: **Weight: Short-term goal =** _____ – _____ = _____ x 3500 = _____ calories	**You need to burn _____ calories over a period of time to lose _____ pounds.**

Formula to learn how many calories of fat we need to scorch for the LONG-term goal!

Exercise A2:

Current weight – **LONG**-term weight goal = Pounds of fat we need to BURN Pounds of fat x 3500 = Amount of calories we need to burn to hit short-term goal	
Candie 200 – 180= **20lbs** **20 x 3500 = 70,000 calories**	**Candie needs to burn 70,000 calories over a period of time to lose 20 pounds.**
Enter your data: **Weight – Short-term goal =** _____ x 3500 = _____	**You need to burn _____ calories over a period of time to lose _____ pounds.**

Now let's find out <u>when</u> you will hit your short- and long-term goals.

Remember, the date is just a target date. It's possible you may hit your goal sooner or a few days or weeks later due to the learning curve in using the A.I.M. Method.

Regardless, you will develop safe, practical, and proven habits for achieving your goal and weight loss management.

This table is based on **losing 1 pound of fat per week or 3,500** calories per week.

Formula to estimate target date for reaching both short- and long-term goals!

Exercise B1

Amount of calories we need to burn to hit **SHORT**-term goal *divided* by 3,500 = weeks needed to hit goal	
Amount of calories we need to burn to hit **LONG**-term goal *divided* by 3,500 = weeks needed to hit goal	
Candie 35,0000 / 3,500 = 10 weeks	**Candie will hit her SHORT-term goal in 10 weeks if she loses 1 pound per week.**
70,000 / 3,500 = 20 weeks	**Candie will hit her LONG-term goal in 20 weeks if she loses 1 pound per week.**

Enter your data: Amount of calories need to burn for short-term goal divided by 3,500 = _____ / 3,500 = Amount of calories need to burn for LONG-term goal divided by 3,500 = _____ / 3,500=	You will hit your SHORT-term goal in _____ weeks if you lose 1 pound per week. You will hit your LONG-term goal in _____ weeks if you lose 1 pound per week.

Online calculator available at www.fitnessfoundy.net

"Abs are made in the kitchen and glutes in the gym."
—Anonymous

You can shorten the time line by choosing to **lose 2 pounds or 7,000** calories per week. I do not recommend using this program to lose more than 2 pounds per week.

Exercise B2

Amount of calories we need to burn to hit **SHORT**-term goal *divided* by 7,000 = weeks needed to hit goal Amount of calories we need to burn to hit **LONG**-term goal *divided* by 7,000 = weeks needed to hit goal	
Candie 35,0000 / 7,000 = 5 weeks 70,000 / 7,000 = 10 weeks	**Candie will hit her SHORT-term goal in 5 weeks if she loses 2 pounds per week.** **Candie will hit her LONG-term goal in 10 weeks if she loses 2 pounds per week.**
Enter your data: **Amount of calories need to burn for short-term goal divided by 7,000** _____ / 7,000 = _____ **Amount of calories need to burn for LONG-term goal divided by 7,000** _____ / 7,000 = _____	**You will hit your SHORT-term goal in _____ weeks if you lose 2 pounds per week.** **You will hit your LONG-term goal in _____ weeks if you lose 2 pounds per week.**

Online calculator available at www.fitnessfoundry.net

This table is based on losing one-half pound of fat per week or 1,750 calories per week. I want to set you up for success. Goals are still 100% achievable.

Exercise B3

Amount of calories we need to burn to hit **SHORT**-term goal *divided* by 1,750 = weeks needed to hit goal Amount of calories we need to burn to hit **LONG**-term goal *divided* by 1,750 = weeks needed to hit goal	
Candie 35,0000 / 1,750 = 20 weeks 70,000 / 1,750 = 40 weeks	**Candie will hit her SHORT-term goal in 20 weeks if she loses ½ pound per week.** **Candie will hit her LONG-term goal in 40 weeks if she loses ½ pound per week.**
Enter your data: **Amount of calories need to burn for short term goal divided by 1,750** _____ / 1,750 = _____ **Amount of calories need to burn for LONG-term goal divided by 3,500 =** _____ / 1,750 = _____	**You will hit your SHORT term goal in _____ weeks if you lose ½ pound per week.** **You will hit your LONG-term goal in _____ weeks if you lose ½ pound per week.**

You are now establishing a realistic timeline to hit your goal and no longer have to do a crash diet or run five miles a day to chip away at your goals.

The timeline is the framework for the **A.I.M. Method.** It shows what to expect each week, and it is the yardstick or gauge for progress.

> **Important:** *Choose what is most realistic for you. Start with one pound. If you are struggling after a few weeks then drop to half a pound. Consistency is very important in developing new habits and long-term results.*

Step 2:

What caloric intake is best for me to hit my goal?

First let's find out if you are you overeating or undereating.

For this section, we need to find out your Basal Metabolic Rate **(BMR)**:

BMR = How many calories are needed for the body to function. Remember, this will be an estimate.

You can also visit www.fitnessfoundry.net and use my online calculators to gather the data.

If you have your current body fat percentage, skip this section and go to Chapter 13 "Katch-McArdle equation."

My preference for obtaining "Basal Metabolic Rate" is with **The Harris-Benedict BMR**. This equation takes into account individual factors such as height, weight, age, and gender.

The Harris-Benedict BMR *(The BMR is a measure for adults only.)*

Women: BMR = 655 + (9.6 x weight in kilos) + (1.8 x height in cm) – (4.7 x age in years)

Men: BMR = 66 + (13.7 x weight in kilos) + (5 x height in cm) – (6.8 x age in years)

Let's use Candie's data to illustrate how to use the Benedict :

- **Age 35, Ht 5' 6" or 167.6 cm*, Current Weight 200 Pounds or 90 Kilos, Body Fat 30%**

- **Use this formula (Height inches x 2.54) to convert your height to centimeters.*

- Exercises 1 to 2 times per week, sedentary lifestyle

- Short term weight loss goal: 190 pounds

- Long term weight loss goal: 180 pounds

Example with Candie's data:

Exercise C

Women: BMR = 655 + (9.6 x weight in kilos) + (1.8 x height in cm) – (4.7 x age in years) Men: BMR = 66 + (13.7 x weight in kilos) + (5 x height in cm) – (6.8 x age in years)	
Using Women BMR = 655 + (9.6 x **90 kilos**) + (1.8 x **167.6 cm**) – (4.7 x **30** years old)	**Candie's BMR = 1,795** calories needed for the body to function. Remember, this will be an estimate.
Select appropriate equation and plug in your data. (From Pg. 17 Questionnaire A) Remember to convert height to cm and weight to kilos.	
	Your BMR = _____ calories needed for the body to function. Remember, this will be an estimate.

Online calculator available at www.fitnessfoundry.net

Once we establish your BMR, we can then compare how many calories you are consuming versus the necessary caloric intake that's conducive to your weight loss goal.

Now let's learn how many calories you need to **MAINTAIN** your **CURRENT** weight. This is also known as your **TDEE** or Total Daily Energy Expenditure.

Simply, multiply your BMR above by this standard Physical Activity Level (**PAL**):

- 1.2 = you are sedentary and do little or no exercise

- 1.375 = you exercise lightly or do a sport 1–3 days/week

- 1.55 = you are moderately active and do exercise or a sport 3–5 days/week

- 1.725 = you are very active with hard exercise or a sport 6–7 days a week

- 1.9 = you are extremely active with very hard exercise or a sport and a physical job or training twice a day

- The general population is at the 1.2 or 1.375 level.

We can use Candie's answers as an example:

- Candie's BMR 1,795 calories and exercises 1 to 2 times per week, sedentary lifestyle

- Candie's physical activity level (PAL) = 1.375 (exercises lightly or does a sport 1–3 days/week)

- Candie's Total Daily Energy Expenditure (TDEE) = 1,795 x 1.375 = 2,468 calories TDEE

SOURCE: Gerrior, Shirley, WenYen Juan, and Basiotis Peter. "An Easy Approach to Calculating Estimated Energy Requirements." Preventing Chronic Disease 3.4 (2006): A129. Print. Website https://www.ncbi.nlm.nih.gov/pmc/articles/PMC1784117/

If Candie does NOT want to lose weight then she can continue to consume up to 2,468 calories daily.

Let's find out your TDEE (Online calculator available at www .fitnessfoundry.net):

Exercise D

Your BMR =	Your PAL =
BMR x PAL = TDEE	
_____ x _____ =	Your TDEE =

Congratulations!

You now know how many calories you may consume if you wish to maintain your CURRENT weight.

Now we can use your current TDEE and create a safe caloric deficit in conjunction with the other steps to help you achieve your weight loss goal.

STOP!

Using the above data, please go to page 108, Bodysculpting Reference Sheet and complete "Part A1, A2, B1"

Here's a typical example of what happens when you do not know how many calories you need to maintain your preferred weight.

Norma, Age 57, Ht 5' 5", Female, Sedentary Full-Time Job, Can Only Commit to Working Out Twice a Week. A few years ago she was 170 pounds; however, with the demands of work and life, her activity decreased and within two years was 30 pounds heavier.

In 2017, she adjusted her weekly goal expectations to meet her schedule's demands and is now equipped to modify her program accordingly.

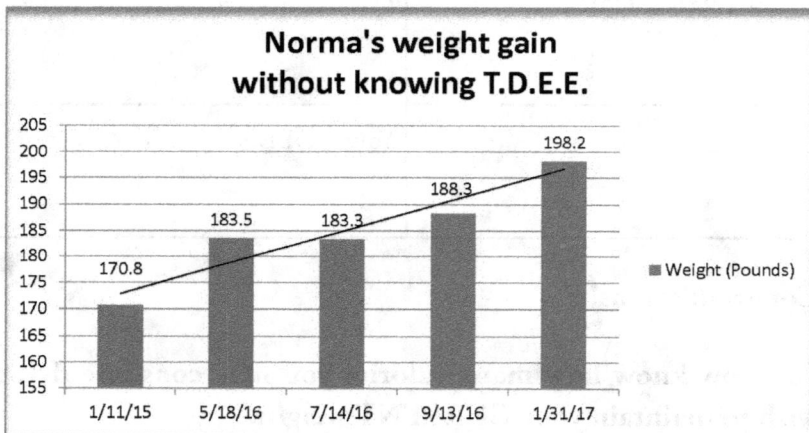

Norma's weight gain without knowing T.D.E.E.

Date	Weight (Pounds)
1/11/15	170.8
5/18/16	183.5
7/14/16	183.3
9/13/16	188.3
1/31/17	198.2

Norma's weight gain could have been prevented by knowing the TDEE she needed to maintain her 170.8 pound weight in 1/15/2015

After 1/31/2017 Norma learned her TDEE and created a realistic sustainable weight loss program that can be adjusted according to her lifestyle.

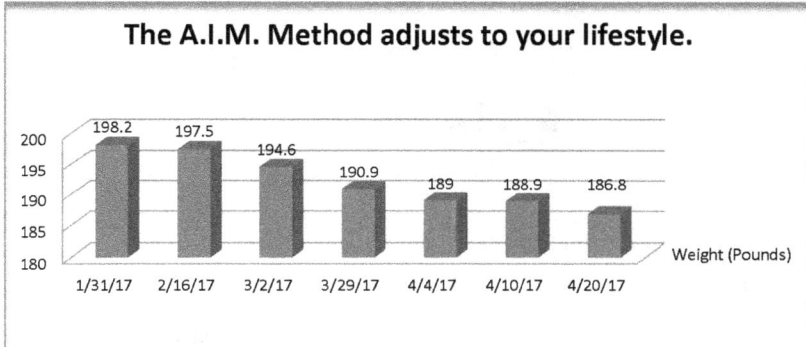

The A.I.M. Method adjusts to your lifestyle.

Date	Weight (Pounds)
1/31/17	198.2
2/16/17	197.5
3/2/17	194.6
3/29/17	190.9
4/4/17	189
4/10/17	188.9
4/20/17	186.8

Norma lost 11.4lbs in just over 2 months!

Get ready! You are now taking your fitness to the NEXT level!

山

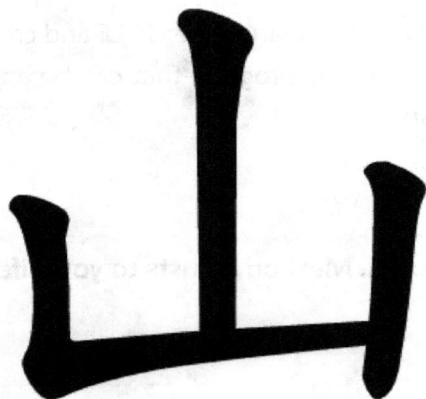

"The greater the obstacle, the more glory in overcoming it."

– MOLIERE

Chapter 4

OPTIMAL CALORIC INTAKE

It's time to shift gears and illustrate how your current TDEE and your answers from the questionnaire will be used to create the foundation of your personalized program.

As we begin to outline your **A.I.M. Method** on a daily and weekly basis, it's important to remember your goal is to hit a deficit of at least 3,500 calories per week.*

* Going forward I will use 3,500 calories to represent a deficit of one pound per week. Please change to 1,750 if you intend to lose half a pound.

The main objective is to identify a specific weight loss goal with a timeline. We will then establish the minimum weekly requirements for the following:

1. Nutrition: Caloric deficit from your TDEE

2. Cardiovascular exercises: Assign an expected caloric expenditure using METs

3. Resistance Training: Assign an expected caloric expenditure using METs

These three modes overlap, and your nutrition deficit will be contingent on how many calories you are scheduled to burn from our cardio and resistance training.

Each mode (nutrition, cardio, resistance training) will be assigned a specific expected caloric expenditure or deficit that that adds up to a weekly total of 3,500 calories required to lose one pound.

METs (Metabolic Equivalent of Tasks) is simply a measurement of how many units of energy is required for the duration of the activity.

* Most fitness and calorie tracking apps have this feature already included.

* For example, walking on the treadmill for 45 minutes at 4 mph for someone who weighs 200 pounds = 330 caloric expenditure/burned (estimate). The MET = 5

I will assist you in learning more on how to find METs for your workouts in the next chapter.

Your weight loss success increases when you move away from obtaining a 3,500 caloric deficit solely from nutrition or excessive cardio.

Reminder: You are training with the purpose of hitting or exceeding a total of 3,500 caloric deficits per week **via the three modes,** not just one mode.

What should my daily caloric intake be to hit my goal?

We will come to this after we establish how many days in the week you can commit to exercising **(From page 17. Questionairre Q1, Q2)**.

We will design a nutrition strategy around your lifestyle and schedule; otherwise your weight loss goal will be too dependent only on your nutrition.

Without understanding how many calories you burn during exercise and not specifically staying within your daily caloric budget is the reason why people **"break even"** as they try to lose weight.

Here's a perfect example:

"I worked out five days during the week but consumed enough calories over the weekend to offset the amount I burned."

This lack of planning will result in a cycle of staying at the same weight or even increasing in overall weight!

Bob, Age 56, Ht 5' 11", Male, Sedentary Job, Full-Time Professional, Travels for Work.

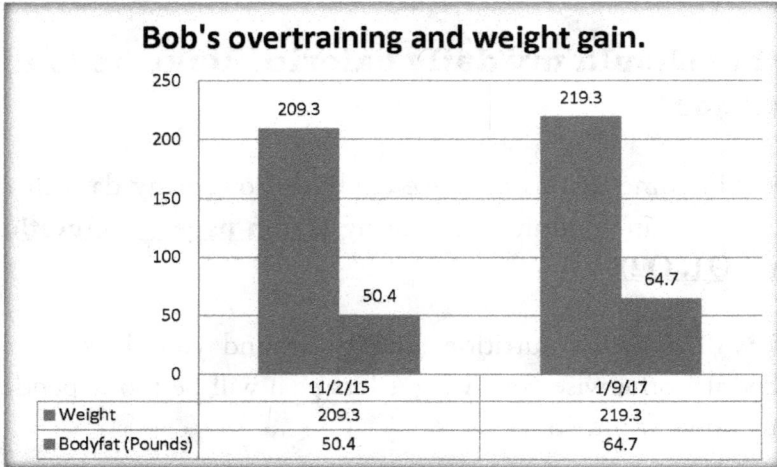

Bob's overtraining and weight gain.

	11/2/15	1/9/17
Weight	209.3	219.3
Bodyfat (Pounds)	50.4	64.7

Prior to using the A.I.M. Method Bob was exercising five days per week, yet gaining weight. In two years he gained 10 pounds. He went from 209 to 219.

Bob overcomes his fitness plateau with The A.I.M. Method.

	1/23/17	1/31/17	2/7/17	2/14/17	2/21/17	3/7/17	4/4/17	4/11/17	4/18/17	4/27/17
■ Weight	217.4	213	215.6	212.1	214.5	214.5	214.5	211.6	213.3	211.9

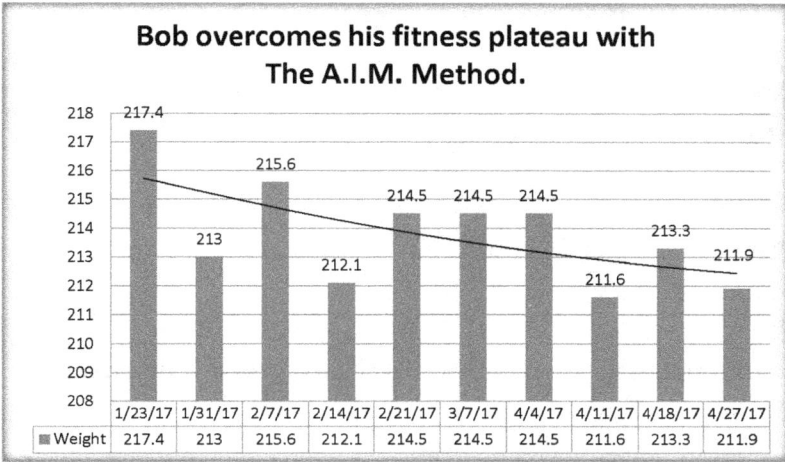

Bob lost the eight pounds of fat he gained in two years in less than four months!

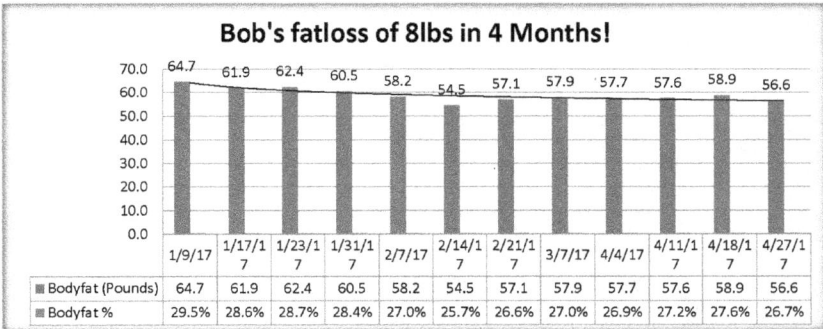

Bob's fatloss of 8lbs in 4 Months!

	1/9/17	1/17/17	1/23/17	1/31/17	2/7/17	2/14/17	2/21/17	3/7/17	4/4/17	4/11/17	4/18/17	4/27/17
■ Bodyfat (Pounds)	64.7	61.9	62.4	60.5	58.2	54.5	57.1	57.9	57.7	57.6	58.9	56.6
■ Bodyfat %	29.5%	28.6%	28.7%	28.4%	27.0%	25.7%	26.6%	27.0%	26.9%	27.2%	27.6%	26.7%

BREAK OUT of breaking even tip:
Be mindful of juice drinks, they are high in sugar!
Avoid the pitfall of drinking your calories!

In this exercise, you will learn how the frequency your workouts directly affects the minimum daily caloric intake you need to hit your goal.

We will use Candie as an example.

Candie can only commit to a 45-minute workout once per week but sometimes can squeeze in twice per week.

Let's presume we assigned an energy expenditure of 310 calories (based on its METs) for Candie's 45-minute treadmill 4 mph workout:

Candie needs to meet or exceed 3,500 calories per week for 1 pound of weight loss.

Candie's Plan A:

- Work out once per week (310 calories burned) and she will need a bigger WEEKLY deficit from her nutrition

- 310 calories burned – 3,500 = 3,190 caloric deficit needed from her weekly nutrition to meet 1 pound of weight loss

Candie's Plan B: Work out twice per week!

- Candie works out twice per week (310 x 2 = 620 calories burned) then she will need a less of a deficit from her nutrition

- 620 calories burned – 3,500 = 2,880 caloric deficit needed from her weekly nutrition to meet 1 pound of weight loss

Candie decided she will use "Plan B" and commit to exercising for 45 minutes twice per week and understands she needs to find a **2,880 caloric deficit from her weekly nutrition** to hit 1 pound of weight loss or 3,500 calories per week.

The next step for Candie is to break down her weekly 2,880 caloric deficit from nutrition to a **daily** amount.

- We simply divide 2,880 by 7 = 412 caloric deficit

- A daily caloric deficit of 412 calories is needed.

Candie now uses her current TDEE from earlier, which is the amount of daily calories she can consume if she does **NOT want to lose weight:** 2,468 calories

- Candie wants to lose weight and can create a customized caloric deficit by deducting 412 from 2,468 (TDEE)

- Candie's suggested DAILY caloric intake to hit her 1 pound a week goal = 2,056 (estimate)

Candie's weekly program to lose 1 pound per week will be the following:

Nutrition: Daily Caloric Intake/Deficit 2,056 / 412 caloric deficit	Nutrition: Weekly Caloric Deficit 412 x 7= 2,884
Resistance Training: Calories burned for duration of session Not Applicable; Candie chooses cardio only	Resistance Training: Weekly Calories Burned N/A
Cardio: Calories burned for duration of session Treadmill 45 minutes 4.0 mph = 310 calories	Cardio: Weekly Calories Burned 310 calories x 2x per week = 620
Weekly Nutrition + Resistance Training + Cardio = 2,884 + 0 + 620 = 3,504! 3,504 calories under her TDEE equals 1 pound of weight loss. She will hit her goal of losing 10 pounds in 10 weeks by losing 1 pound per week!	

Without the tools to show how close she is to burning 3,500 calories she may have skipped a workout and continued the cycle of **not seeing results.**

Candie is NO longer "breaking even"!

Important note:

As I mentioned earlier, Candie can shorten her time line to reaching her goals by committing to lose two pounds per week; however, for her lifestyle it would **NOT be realistic.** She can also drop her weekly weight loss goal to half a pound weekly if nutrition is challenging.

Her progress will be steady, and reaching her goal on the target date is contingent on her consistency, discipline, and outside support.

Main takeaway from Candie's example:

- The more frequent your weekly workouts, the less caloric deficit you will need from your nutrition.

- Your program needs to be realistic and based on your current lifestyle.

- The A.I.M. Method can be adjusted to your lifestyle and frequency of activities.

- You can now choose to lose half, one pound, or even two pounds per week!

- It's time to "BREAK OUT of breaking even"!

Now it's your turn! In Chapter 5 we will personalize *YOUR* program!

山

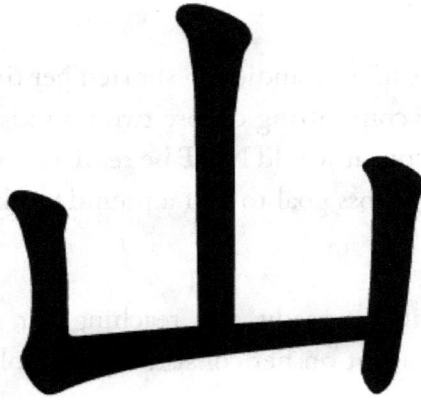

"It does not matter how slowly you go as long as you do not stop."

— CONFUCIUS

Chapter 5

HOW TO TRAIN WITH A PURPOSE

The frequency of your weekly **cardio** and **resistance training** will come from your answers to Question 1 and 2 from Questionnaire A.

Please note your answers . . .

Q1. How many days per week can you REALISTICALLY work out?	Answer:
Q2. What is the duration of your workout?	Answer:

Q3. How many days per week can you realistically do resistance training?	Answer:
Q4. What is the duration of your resistance training?	Answer:
Q3. How many days per week can you realistically do cardio?	Answer:
Q4. What is the duration of your cardio workout? List the equipment(s).	Answer:

The key word in the question 1 is **_REALISTICALLY_**. You do not want to set yourself up for failure.

Once we establish how often you will work out, we can then get an estimate of how many calories you will burn for the cardio or workout session. We get this data by using the Metabolic Equivalent of Tasks or **METs**.

Fun Fact: To find out how much energy/calories you burn at rest use this formula: 1 METs = 3.5 x weight in kg

Brief explanation about METs (Metabolic Equivalent of Tasks) is simply a measurement of how many units of energy is required for the duration of the activity.

- Most fitness and calorie tracking apps have this feature already included.

- For example, walking on the treadmill for 45 minutes at 4 mph for someone who weighs 200 pounds = 330 caloric expenditure/burned (estimate). Its MET = 5

Links for a library of activities that show METs (2011 Compendium of Physical Activities):

- https://www.ncbi.nlm.nih.gov/pubmed/21681120

- http://www.juststand.org/Portals/3/literature/compendium-of-physical-activities.pdf

Use this formula to learn how the caloric expenditure for each activity is calculated. (Most are included in fitness/calorie tracking apps, online calculators, or go to www.fitnessfoundry.net)

METs x Weight (kg) x Time= Calories

The calculation only works with weight in kilograms. To get kilograms from pounds, divide pounds by .45 The calculation also requires that time be in hours. If the activity is only 15 minutes, you would use .25 hours. Formula to convert to hours = Time/60

For example, to estimate how many calories a 150 pound (~70 kg) person would burn during 30 minutes of gardening (5 METs), use the calculation below:

Calories burned = 5 x 68.2 kg x .5 hour = 170.5 calories

(http://www.mhhe.com/hper/physed/clw/webreview/web07/tsld007.htm)

Important! Use the table below to outline your cardio and resistance training caloric expenditure:

Exercise E1

Name of Exercise	METS (use formula)	Duration	Calories burned (using formula)	How often during the week?	Total weekly calories burned
Treadmill	5	45 minutes	310	2	620
Add up "Total Weekly Calories Burned" for all exercises (answer will be used in next section).					

Alternatives to doing the math yourself:

1. Some fitness/calorie tracking apps have this included

2. You may use online calculators

3. Go to www.fitnessfoundry.net

Next Step: Exercise E2

We need to find out how much of a **weekly caloric deficit from nutrition** is needed to hit 1 pound of weight loss per week or 3,500 calories.

"Total of weekly calories burned" – 3,500 = _____ (weekly caloric deficit needed from nutrition)

Use the following equations: **Use answer from Exercise E1, Pg. 46**

_____ – 3,500 = _____ (weekly caloric deficit needed from nutrition)

Divide your "weekly caloric deficit needed from nutrition" by 7:

Now we can find out your "daily caloric deficit."

_____ / 7 = _____ (daily caloric deficit)

("A" use answer for next section)

Finally, we can find your suggested caloric intake that's conducive to your goal.

You will need your TDEE from earlier:

Your TDEE – Daily caloric deficit = _____ (daily caloric intake to hit goal) (From Pg. 29)

_____ – _____ = daily caloric intake to hit goal (**"B" use answer for next section**)

As a reminder, we are training with purpose of hitting or exceeding a total of 3,500 caloric deficits per week **via nutrition, cardio, and resistance training,** not just one mode.

Let's find out if you will "BREAK OUT of breaking even"!

Exercise F
(Use "A" and "B" Answers from Previous Questions)

Nutrition: Daily Caloric Intake/ Deficit
   "B"   "A"
    /   caloric deficit
	Nutrition: Weekly Caloric Deficit
	"A" x 7 =

Resistance Training: Calories burned for duration of session	Resistance Training: Weekly Calories Burned *Multiply Answer x Number of Days*
Cardio: Calories burned for duration of session	Cardio: Weekly Calories Burned *Multiply Answer x Number of Days*

Weekly Nutrition + Resistance Training + Cardio = 3,500 or more	
+	
+ =	

Online calculator available at www.fitnessfoundry.net

The personalized combination of weekly nutrition, resistance train-ing, and cardio will equal a 3,500 calorie deficit. Knowing the assigned expenditure for each mode will help in planning your week.

You will NO longer be "breaking even"!

Jane, Age 48, Ht 5' 5", Female, Professional

From 7/16/2016–1/5/2017 she was "breaking even" despite working out five times per week.

Jane's results prior to using A.I.M Method.

	7/18/16	1/5/17
Weight	146.8	148.7
Bodyfat (Pounds)	43.0	44.5

Since 1/5/2017 with the A.I.M. Method Jane was able to commit to ½ pound per week of weight loss, which was sustainable and realistic for her lifestyle.

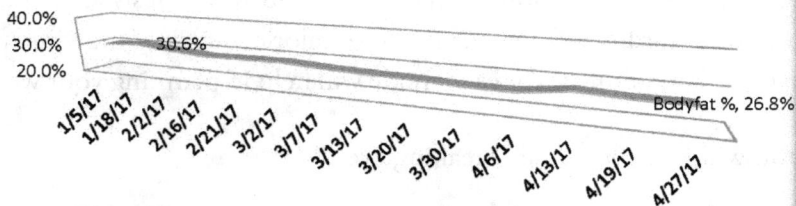

½ lb per week of weight loss was most realistic for Jane's lifestyle. She experienced a decrease of 3% bodyfat in 4 months.

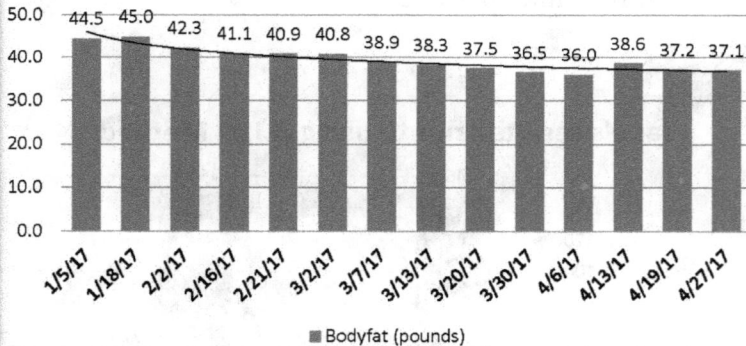

Jane lost 7lbs of bodyfat after using The A.I.M. Method in 4 months!

Important note:

As I mentioned earlier, you can shorten your time line by committing to lose two pounds per week; however, make sure it is **realistic** for your lifestyle.

Main takeaways:

- The more frequent your weekly workouts, the less caloric deficit you will need from your nutrition.

- Your program needs to be realistic and based on your current lifestyle.

- The **A.I.M. Method** can be adjusted to your lifestyle and frequency of activities.

- You can now choose to lose one pound or even two pounds per week!

- It's time to "BREAK OUT of breaking even"!

STOP!

Using the above data, please go to page 108, Bodysculpting Reference Sheet and complete "Part B2, C"

山

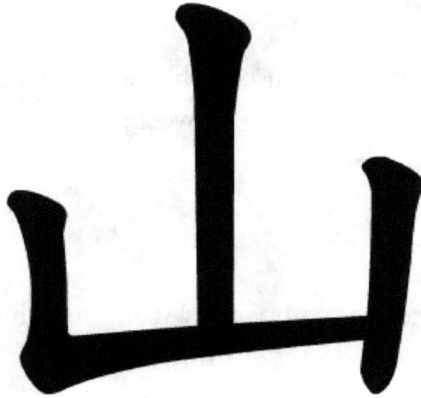

"Great works are performed not by strength but by perseverance."

— SAMUEL JOHNSON

Chapter 6

INITIATE: HOW TO MAXIMIZE YOUR TIME AND EFFORTS

Phew! Now that you have done the math, it's time to put your plans into action!

It's important to remember, similar to other endeavors, learning from your experience and continued practice will lead to confidence and better results!

Weekly Nutrition + Resistance Training + Cardio = 3,500 or more (Answers from Exercise F, page 49)

+   +   =

We now have your daily and weekly caloric intake:

_____

You have committed to X days for weekly workouts:

_____

We now have the duration and how many calories you need to burn per workout . _____

I highly suggest partnering with a friend or gym buddy and starting this journey together.

Your results may come easier when you have someone to share your challenges and successes.

Now it's time for practical tips for **exercise selection**.

This section will outline common low impact exercises that yield the most caloric expenditure in the shortest amount of time.

In the previous questionnaire I asked why you exercised or did cardio and if it was specifically for weight loss. Review your answers and let's select exercises that have the SOLE purpose of maximizing your caloric expenditure in the same or less amount of time.

Remember METs and its relationship to intensity.

Here we'll use Candie as an example:

Candie can only commit to a 45-minute workout one time per week but sometimes can squeeze in two times per week.

We assigned an energy expenditure of 310 calories based on 5 METs for a vigorous resistance workout for Candie's 45-minute workout:

She does a resistance workout with free weights doing compound lifts and working big muscles.

Here's a simple comparison of other exercises she could do for 45 minutes that would either be under or over her caloric goal.

We are trying to maximize her time and insure it's conducive to burning 310 calories per workout.

> Just a reminder: She already has a planned weekly caloric deficit from nutrition of 2,884 and needs to reach 3,500 for 1 pound of weight loss per week.

The remaining calories will come from exercising; the minimum she needs to burn is 310 calories per workout (estimate). If done twice in the week (620 calories) would meet the difference needed to add up to 3,500 calories.

Exercise	METs with requirements	Calories burned for 45 minutes	Does it meet/ exceed 310 calories?
Free weight Training	5 METs vigorous	310 calories burned	Yes
Group Exercise	7.8 METs	526 calories burned	Yes; exceeds
Treadmill	3 METs, 2.5 mph No incline	202 calories burned	No
Treadmill	5 METs, 4 mph	330 calories burned	Yes; exceeds
Yoga	Type ranges from 2.5 METs to 4 METs	Max 270 calories burned	No
Golf	Walking, carrying clubs 4.5 METs	303 calories burned	No
Running	4 mph, 13 min/ mile, 6 METs	405 calories burned	Yes; exceeds
Spinning	100–160 watts, 8.8 METs	594 calories burned	Yes; exceeds

METs from http://www.juststand.org/Portals/3/literature/compendium-of-physical-activities.pdf

Here are my suggestions for exercises for a variety of schedules:

The A.I.M. Method has 2 cycles with 12-week micro cycles (estimated weeks to hit short-term goal)

Cycle 1: Exercise prescription until **short**-term goal is reached. After 12 weeks, reassess successes and challenges. Modify the next 12 weeks according to previous micro cycle.

Cycle 2: Exercise prescription until **long**-term goal is reached. After 12 weeks, reassess successes and challenges. Modify next 12 weeks according to previous micro cycle.

Chart B

Frequency of weekly exercise availability	Frequency of Resistance Training	Frequency of Cardio	Resistance/ Cardio
		Cycle 1	Cycle 2
You can go 1x per week	N/A	1x for 55 minutes	Same
You can go 2x per week	1x for 55 minute (10 minutes warmup)	1x for 55 minutes	Same
You can go 3x per week	1x for 55 minute (10 minutes warmup)	2x for 55 minutes	2x/1x
You can go 4x per week	2x for 55 minute (10 minutes warmup)	2x for 55 minutes	3x/1x
You can go 5x per week	2x for 55 minute (10 minutes warmup)	3x for 55 minutes	3x/2x

Frequency of weekly exercise availability	Frequency of Resistance Training	Frequency of Cardio	Resistance/ Cardio
You can go 6x per week	2x for 55 minute (10 minutes warmup)	4x for 55 minutes	4x/2x
You can go 7x per week	You are . . .	over- . . .	training!

Please review your exercise selection to see if it is the most efficient and meets necessary caloric expenditure for the workout.

Planned weekly caloric deficit from nutrition (from pg. 49 Exercise F):_____.   _____

Your required caloric expenditure per workout (pg. 46).
_____ Total for week_____.

Do they add up to 3,500 for 1 pound of weight loss per week or more?*

Remember: You can lower your caloric deficit to 1,750 or ½ pound if you find a 3,500 calorie deficit too difficult to meet consistently.

Review the following list to determine the most effective exercises to choose for calorie burning and time efficiency. Using the METS formula we reviewed earlier (page 45), you can calculate the number of calories burned in the session

1. Use this formula to learn how the caloric expenditure for each activity (some fitness/calorie tracking apps have this included, use online calculators, or go to www.fitnessfoundry.net

METs x Weight (kg) x Time = Calories

The calculation only works with weight in kilograms. To get kilograms from pounds divide pounds by .45 The calculation also requires that time be in hours. If the activity is only 15 minutes, you would use .25 hours.

Also, most apps will be able to give you an estimate for resistance workouts, but it's good to double-check with our calculation. Using a heart rate monitor will give approximate data on the caloric expenditure.

Exercise G
(See Candie's Example Page 56)

Exercise	METs with requirements	Calories burned for minutes	Does it meet/exceed calories?
Enter your realistic duration of time to exercise and compare caloric expenditure. Most common exercises: Add your own and include required intensity and METs			
Free weight Training	5 METs, vigorous		
Group Exercise	7.8 METs		
Treadmill	3 METs, 2.5 mph No incline		
Treadmill	5 METs, 4 mph		

Exercise	METs with requirements	Calories burned for minutes	Does it meet/exceed calories?
Yoga	Type ranges from 2.5 METs to 4 METs		
Golf	Walking, carrying clubs 4.5 METs		
Running	4 mph, 13 min/mile, 6 METs		
Spin	100–160 watts, 8.8 METs		
Rowing	100 watts, 7 METs		
Elliptical	Moderate, 5 METs		

Choose the equipment/modality that has the maximum amount of caloric expenditure.

Find other exercises/activities such as:

- Versaclimber

- hiking

- arc trainer

- elliptical

- swimming

- rowing

- cycling

- walking

- stepmill

Links for a library of activities that show METs:

- https://www.ncbi.nlm.nih.gov/pubmed/21681120

- http://www.juststand.org/Portals/3/literature/compendium-of-physical-activities.pdf

- www.fitnessfoundry.net

I highly suggest keeping your exercises low impact. This program is designed for weight loss not for sport performance.

Use discretion when choosing running or high impact exercises and ask yourself if the risks are worth the benefits. Far too often individuals are sidelined from physical activities due to unnecessary high-impact exercises when their primary goal was to lose weight.

Return to high-impact activities after you hit your weight loss goal!

The balance of cardio and resistance training would be based on my suggestion from chart B page 57.

Strength training is a key component for long-term weight management, and cardio is also essential to burn the fat among other health benefits.

Both have a specific role and designated place for each cycle to optimize your results. So please: Follow the instructions!

STOP!

Using the above data, please go to page 108, Bodysculpting Reference Sheet and complete "Part C"

山

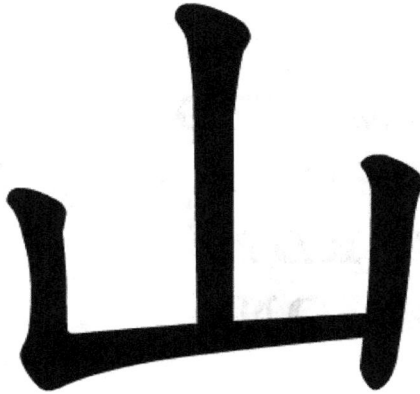

*"I've always been an underdog.
I feel like I beat the odds."*
– J. COLE

Chapter 7

CUSTOMIZED RESISTANCE TRAINING AND CARDIO SELECTION

Why Resistance Training? To increase metabolism, to gain muscle memory and functional strength, to spare muscle, preserve joint integrity, and lay the groundwork for body sculpting after completion of Cycle 2.

If your workout has the appropriate intensity, you will continue to burn calories up to 72 hours post workout.

Resistance training basics for both cycles: *Change exercise selection/circuit every six to nine weeks!*

- 2–4 circuits of exercises that end at 55 minutes or less but hit the necessary caloric expenditure

- 1 circuit may have 3–5 exercises. It's important to go from one exercise to the other with no more than two minutes of rest. The less rest time the better, but use discretion to avoid overexertion or injury.

- 12–15 Reps and 4 sets for 55-minute workouts including 10 minute warmups

Tips for exercises and workouts: *Exercise more muscle per movement to burn more calories!*

- Perform total body exercises that include resistance such as thrusters, squats variations, step ups, push and pull exercises, battle ropes, sled

- Limit your seated exercises to 1 per workout, e.g. lat seated cable row

- Compound lifts: squats, dead lifts

- Work biggest muscles: quadriceps, hamstrings, chest, back, shoulders

- Body weight exercises such as planks can be added but should be only one exercise out of the circuit. Abdominal exercises should be done AFTER your workout is completed.

- If you complete all the sets and complete all the repetitions, then you MUST go up in weight for your next workout, e.g. increments of 2.5 pounds

- This is called progressive overload: As you continue to lose weight, your strength will increase with time.

- Always have an assigned caloric expenditure for the duration of the workout.

Preference of equipment:

- Freeweights, barbells, kettlebells, cable cross

- Machines (preferably use at the end of a workout), medicine balls, resistance tubes

- Exception for resistance training: If you find that bodyweight exercises meet the caloric expenditure for your workout as it's required for you to hit goal then please do the bodyweight exercises. A heart rate monitor can establish how many calories you are burning.

- Refer to page 59 Exercise G for exercises that have optimal caloric expenditure.

Why not only do cardio? You want to spare muscle. You are working toward long-term weight management, building strong muscles, and improving joint integrity to allow you to stay active for years to come.

Cardio training basics for phase both cycles:

- Have two cardio selections. Both should have the minimum caloric expenditure.

- Pair cardio exercises together; for example, 20 minutes walking on treadmill, then 15 minutes rowing.

- Use cardio equipment that recruits more muscles per movement, e.g. rowing, arc trainer, swimming

- The more muscles you use, the more calories you burn.

- You can always do a split cardio day, such as training for 30 minutes in the morning, and returning in the evening for an additional 30 minutes.

- Change the type of cardio you do every six to nine weeks, but maintain or increase caloric expenditure.

- Remember: You are doing cardio for weight loss, not performance. Stay focused on intensity and time.

Preference of equipment:

- jump rope

- Versaclimber

- arc trainer

- step mill

- rowing

- spin bike

- treadmill

- swimming

Always have an assigned caloric expenditure for the duration of your workout.

Refer to page 59, Exercise G for exercises that have optimal caloric expenditure.

Below you will find the benefits of using METs to identify the best exercises solely for weight loss rather than sport performance results.

- Jonas, Age 42, Ht 6', 183 cm,* Start Weight 229 Pounds, 103 Kilos, Body Fat 21.8%

- *Use this formula (Height inches x 2.54) to convert your height to centimeters.

- Exercises up to five times per week, active lifestyle

- Short-term weight loss goal: 204 pounds

- Long-term weight loss goal: Body fat 12%

Jonas was not maximizing his workout time for weight loss. Rather, he was focusing on strength. Then he changed his exercise selection along with reps and sets to meet the caloric expenditure. This was paired up with a personalized sustainable nutrition plan with the best macros for him based on his body type.

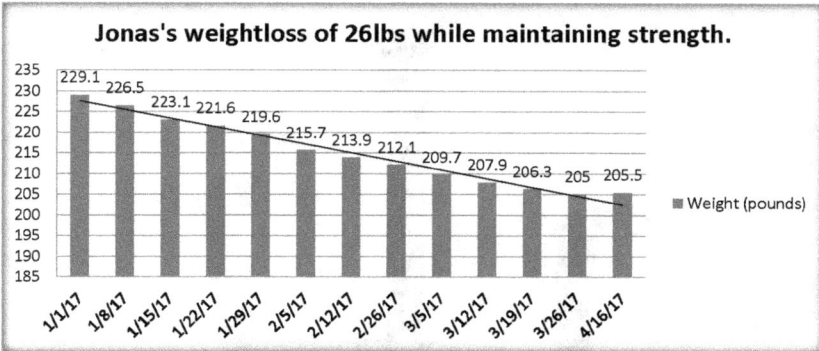

Jonas's weightloss of 26lbs while maintaining strength.

His short-term goal of 204 pounds was not hit on the 12th week/"target date," but you can see he was trending in the right direction!

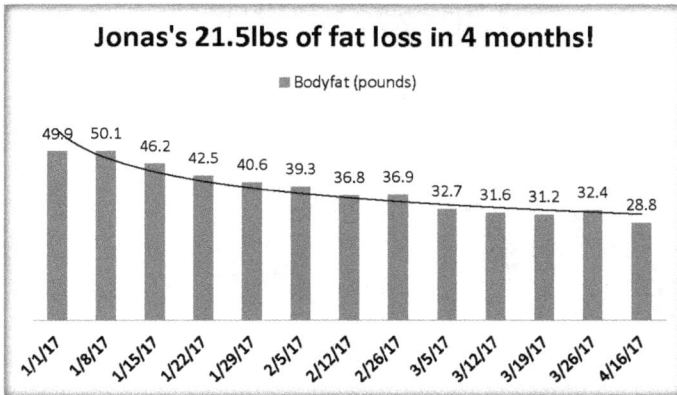

Jonas's 21.5lbs of fat loss in 4 months!

Over the 12 weeks, Jonas made lifestyle changes conducive to his goal and became healthier.

Now he focuses on his macros and updates his **A.I.M. Method** to match his 12% body fat goal.

Congratulations! You now have the tools to get started. Now we are going to fine tune YOUR program.

山

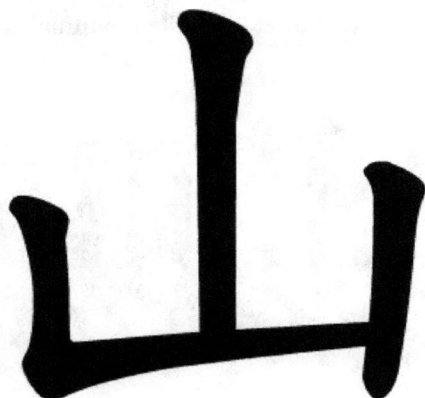

"No! Try not! Do or DO NOT!
There is no 'try.'"

— YODA

Chapter 8

NUTRITION: THE KEY TO NOT "BREAKING EVEN"

If diets worked, then the vast majority of people would be at their ideal weight.

When you are working toward a weight loss goal, the caloric deficit needs to realistic and sustainable for the time needed to reach the weight loss goal.

Four factors that will personalize your caloric budget and help you reach your goal:

1. Knowing your TDEE or how many calories you can consume to maintain your current weight will set the baseline. We established this earlier with Exercise D pg. 29.

2. Determining how often you can exercise for the week will dictate the remaining calories needed to reach a deficit of 3,500 calories per week. We established this with Exercise E2 pg. 47.

3. Using the difference from the amount of caloric expenditure from exercises and subtracting it from calories to maintain will give you your daily and weekly caloric budget. Exercise E1 pg. 46.

4. Avoid the misperception that you can eat more because you worked out more. This will not only keep you from seeing results, but perpetuate the cycle of rollercoaster weight gain/loss and "breaking even."

The above will give us a caloric budget that is truly personalized to your lifestyle.

Not having set a total weekly caloric deficit and not tracking is a recipe for "breaking even."

They work hand in hand.

Let me illustrate a typical scenario.

Candie's example:

Her daily deficit from nutrition is 412 calories. This adds up to a weekly total of 2,884 calories. Her weekly total deficit will increase if she eats less than her daily caloric budget.

Going above the daily caloric budget may lead to "breaking even;" she will only be replacing the calories she burned from her activities by eating.

Candie's weekly calories need to be under 14,392, otherwise she may "break even" even with her workouts.

Assume she has not missed her workouts and was hitting the appropriate intensity to reach a 310 caloric expenditure per workout. She works out two times per week.

Her progress was stymied by the extra carbohydrates and high caloric beverages from a work event in week 3.

Fun fact: Did you know that alcohol provides 7 calories per gram, second to fat 9 calories, carbs and protein 4 calories per gram.

Takeaways from Candie's "break even" example:

- Look for trends in nutrition, cardio, exercise that are not conducive to your goals.

- **IMPORTANT!** Every seven days, weigh in and add up the weekly numbers. This is very important to see why you are breaking even, and it holds YOU accountable.

- There is a learning curve!

- By reviewing her numbers, Candie was made conscious of what she was eating, the caloric density, and whether she wanted to "break even" again.

- When you get closer to the seventh day of tracking you can adjust your activity or food intake to hit your weekly goal.

Candie	Mon	Tues	Weds	Thurs	Fri	Sat	Sun	Expected Weekly Calories from Nutrition	Difference Between Expect Weekly Calories and Actual	Total Weekly Caloric Deficit	Expected Weekly Calories from Exercise	Expected Weekly Total Calories	How many lost pounds Per Week
Budget	2056	2056	2056	2056	2056	2056	2056	14,392	0	2884	620	3504	1 pound
Week 1	2100	1900	2250	2000	1800	2120	2100	14,270	Under 122	2884 + 112 = 2996	620	3616	1 pound+
Week 2	2100	1900	2350	2000	1800	2120	2100	14,370	Under 22	2884 + 22 = 2906	620	3616	1 pound
Week 3	*2450*	*1900*	*2250*	*2000*	*2100*	*2220*	*2300*	*15,320*	*Over 950*	*2884– 950 = 1934*	*620*	*2554*	½ pound

- More importantly, even if you do not hit your weekly goal this does NOT mean you will not meet your weight loss goal.

- You are learning how to use tools that give you control over your weight.

- Continued practice makes progress not perfection!

- Losing weight for the long term is a process.

- Learn to identify foods that need to be replaced or portion controlled.

- Use weeks of "breaking even" for vacations and other special occasions.

Many of us are gung ho in the beginning but start to fizzle out or become complacent after 21 days.

Habits are generally formed after 90 days, so it's more important to stay consistent rather than striving for perfection.

One huge benefit of tracking is the subtle development of a new lifestyle that's realistic and conducive to achieving goals.

山

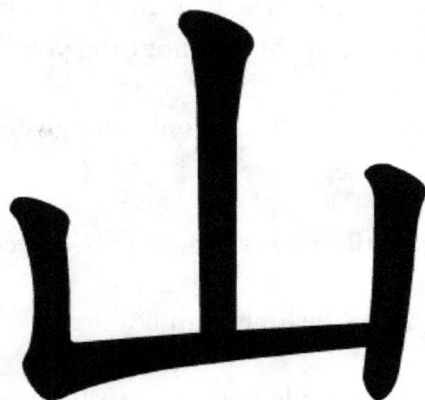

"The great victory, which appears so simple today, was a series of small victories gone unnoticed."
—Paolo Coelho

Chapter 9

NON-NEGOTIABLES FOR WEIGHT LOSS: MACROS AND TIPS FROM PEERS

"Non-negotiables" for weight loss may sound restrictive, but you need parameters that will keep you on the road to success.

Weight loss is achieved simply by sticking to an assigned caloric deficit for a period of time until you hit your target weight.

As you lose weight, you will be able to refine your nutrition with timing, macronutrients, and supplements along with expanding your exercise selection.

What are macronutrients?

Protein = 4 calories per gram, Carbohydrates = 4 calories per gram, and Fat = 9 calories per gram.

Here are some tips on how to personalize your nutrition by identifying your body type:

Set your macronutrient by choosing one of these three body types (somatotype)

It is not an exact science, but it will give you a sound start on deciding which are the best macronutrients for you:

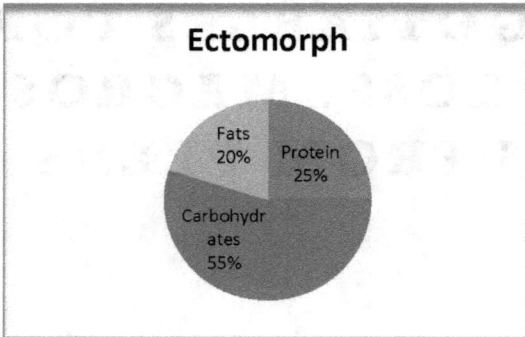

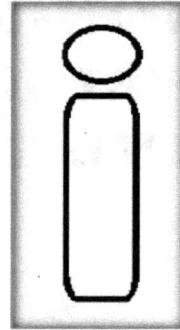

- Ectomorph: Fast metabolic rate. Thin build with longer limbs and a high tolerance for carbohydrates. A good starting macronutrient ratio for you would be 25% protein, 55% carbs, and 20% fat.

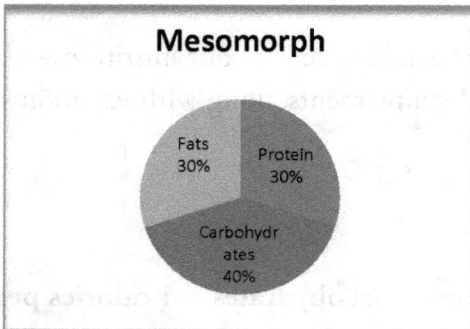

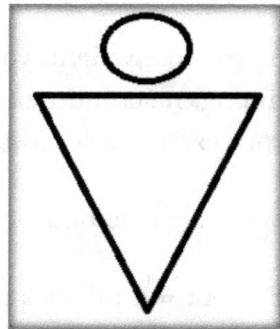

- Mesomorph: They have muscular build with narrow waist. Moderate carbohydrate tolerance and a moderate metabolic rate. Important to note, may gain fat more easily than ectomorphs. Mesomorphs can usually start at a 30% protein, 40% carbs, 30% fat macronutrient ratio.

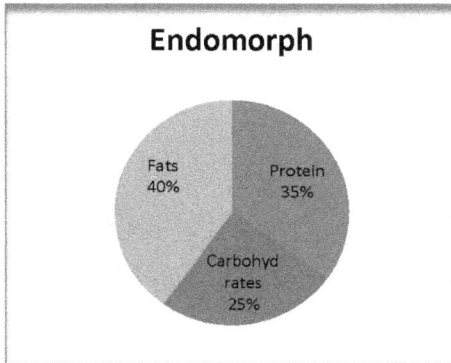

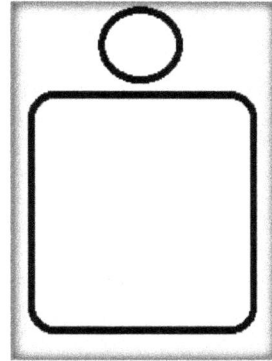

- Endomorph: They have a more blocky build with hips as wide as clavicles and shorter limbs. Low carbohydrate tolerance and a slow metabolic rate. They tend to store more body fat and find it hard to lose fat. If you're an endomorph, try a ratio of 35% protein, 25% carbs, and 40% fat.

- It's possible to have characteristics from different body types. This is a generalization of body types.

SOURCE: Dietary Reference Intakes for Energy, Carbohydrate. Fiber, Fat, Fatty Acids, Cholesterol, Protein, and Amino Acids (2002/2005).

This report may be accessed via www.nap.edu

During the process of weight loss, your body will lose both fat and muscle. You will minimize muscle waste by exercising and consuming an adequate amount of protein.

Here are some healthy choices from each macro category:

Proteins

- Complete proteins are found in animal sources. Meat (poultry, fish, pork, red meat), eggs, and dairy products including whole milk, cottage cheese, and milk protein powders (casein and whey)

- Vegetarians: You may also get protein from plants, e.g. grains, seeds, lentils, soybeans, tofu

Carbohydrates: There are three types of carbohydrates, simple, complex and fiber.

- Simple carbohydrates come from various forms of sugar, such as sucrose (table sugar), fructose (fruit sugars), lactose (dairy sugar), and glucose (blood sugar). Minimize consumption of simple carbs, e.g. sports drinks, candy, breads, etc.

- Complex carbs come from vegetables and unrefined whole grains. These make you feel fuller and digest slowly and include potatoes, casava, greens, unrefined oatmeal, unrefined oat bran, and legumes (beans).

- Fiber can have a significant effect on weight loss. High fibrous foods include edamame, avocado, broccoli, pears (with skin), bran, various legumes, artichokes, and greens.

"The glycemic index ranks carbohydrates on a scale from 0 to 100 based on how quickly and how much they raise blood sugar levels after eating. Foods with a high glycemic index, like white bread, are rapidly digested and cause substantial fluctuations in blood sugar. Foods with a low glycemic index, like whole oats, are digested more slowly, prompting a more gradual rise in blood sugar."

https://www.hsph.harvard.edu/nutritionsource/carbohydrates/carbohydrates-and-blood-sugar/

Fats: There are three types of fats:

- saturated (butter, animal fats, tropical oils like coconut and palm kernel),

- mono-unsaturated (avocado, olive oil, peanuts, almonds, pecans)

- poly-unsaturated (Omega-3/Omega-6, fish, flaxseed, canola, safflower). You'll want to get the majority of your fats from the unsaturated categories.

It's important to note that your caloric budget is non-negotiable. How you set up your macros will assist in retaining muscle, energy, metabolism, and optimizing your body's performance during the process of weight loss.

If you decided to incorporate Intermittent fasting then be sure to have set macros to prevent muscle loss.

Arthur, Age 40, Male, Ht 6', Active Lifestyle,

Works from Home, Two Young Children, Works Out 1x Per Week.

Arthur's food selection was very healthy; however his macros were high in calories, which offset his once a week workout. With the A.I.M. method, he was able to create a sustainable and realistic program for his lifestyle.

Prior to 1/5/2017 Arthur's strategy for losing weight was to have a significant caloric deficit, which started a cycle of rollercoaster weight loss and gain.

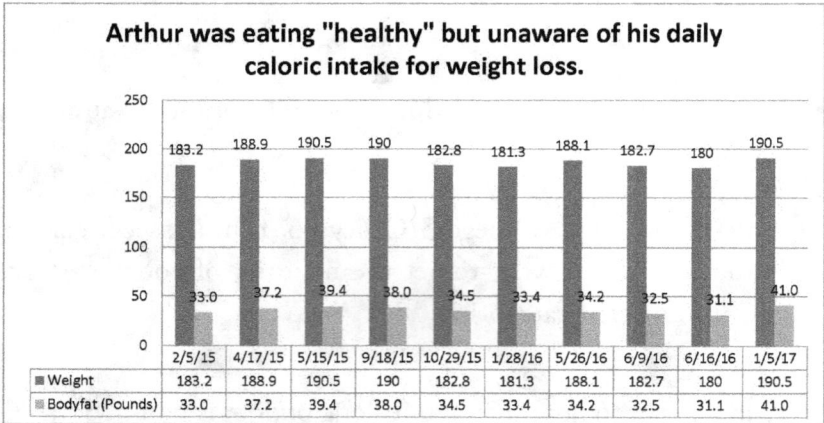

Arthur was eating "healthy" but unaware of his daily caloric intake for weight loss.

	2/5/15	4/17/15	5/15/15	9/18/15	10/29/15	1/28/16	5/26/16	6/9/16	6/16/16	1/5/17
Weight	183.2	188.9	190.5	190	182.8	181.3	188.1	182.7	180	190.5
Bodyfat (Pounds)	33.0	37.2	39.4	38.0	34.5	33.4	34.2	32.5	31.1	41.0

After 1/5/2017 Arthur used the A.I.M. Method to create a realistic nutrition plan with a large caloric deficit. He also assigned a caloric expenditure to his weekly workout.

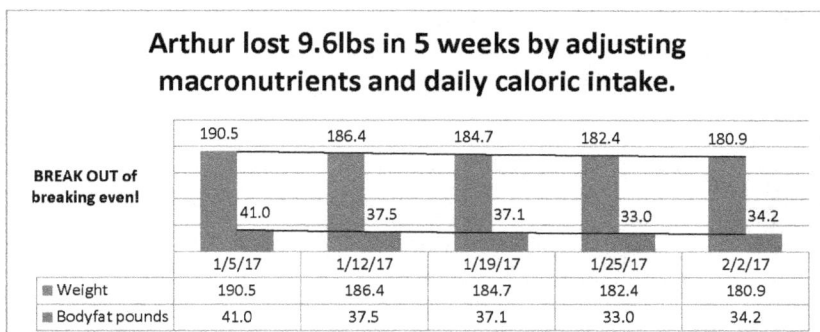

Arthur lost 9.6lbs in 5 weeks by adjusting macronutrients and daily caloric intake.

BREAK OUT of breaking even!	1/5/17	1/12/17	1/19/17	1/25/17	2/2/17
■ Weight	190.5	186.4	184.7	182.4	180.9
■ Bodyfat pounds	41.0	37.5	37.1	33.0	34.2

There are many brands of diets, weight loss systems, and exercise programs that will speak of losing XX amount of weight. They all have the same formula. It's a caloric deficit for a period of time.

- The **main** non-negotiable is that you have a weekly caloric deficit.

- Low glycemic foods will assist in stabilizing insulin.

- Consistency with the suggestions (even if you are not hitting your daily goals) and time will lead to improvement.

The **A.I.M. Method** is designed to give you tools to have total control of how much weight you want to lose based on your lifestyle. It's not based on a one-size-fits-all diet, deprivation, or requiring an excessive unsustainable amount of weekly workouts that might lead to injuries.

Here are real world tips from other people who are using the **A.I.M. Method**:

- Suggest only tracking carbohydrates and protein for the first few weeks in Cycle 1.

- Identify alternatives to high caloric foods and drinks.

- Sometimes changing the portion lets you enjoy comfort foods and beverages, too.

- Stay vigilant over the weekend.

- Iced coffee nutrition example: using one cream instead of two cuts calories in half.

- Identify boredom and stress eating and overcome with low glycemic foods.

- Combine protein meals with foods with enzymes, e.g. papaya, pineapple

- Consume raw veggies as snacks, e.g. bell peppers, celery

STOP!

Using the above data, please go to page 108, Bodysculpting Reference Sheet and complete "Part B3"

山

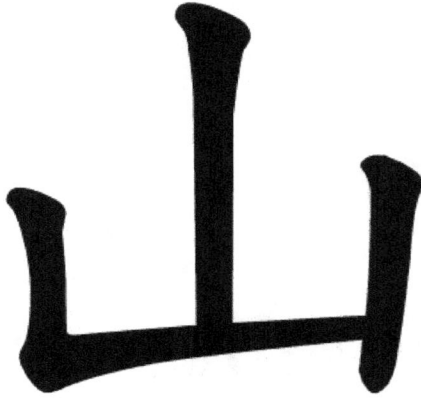

"To rally every black sheep is my goal."
— JULIAN COPE

Chapter 10

MOTIVATION: MINIMIZING CHALLENGES AND TIPS ON MAINTENANCE

Losing weight is not a linear process, and you can expect bumps in the road. However, you can minimize the rollercoaster by looking for trends, and this is done by tracking your caloric intake and expenditure.

Candie	Expected Weekly Calories from Nutrition	Difference Between Expect Weekly Calories and Actual	Total Weekly Caloric Deficit	Expected Weekly Calories from Exercise	Expected Weekly Total Calories	How Many Pounds Per Week	Weight	New Weight
Needed	14,392	0	2884	620	3504	1 pound		200
Week 1	14,270	Under 122	2884 + 112 = 2996	620	3616	1+ pound		199
Week 2	14,370	Under 22	2884 + 22 = 2906	620	3616	1 pound		198
Week 3	*15,320*	*Over 950*	*2884 – 950 = 1934*	*620*	*2554*	*½ + pound*		*197.5*

We can see a dip in Candie's weekly total loss of weight in week three. That week there may have been an event that lead her to eat more.

Here are some common experiences for Cycle 1, Weeks 1–12:

Weeks 1 to 3

- You may find tracking your food challenging for the first week.

- You can find general caloric estimates from online or food apps for many restaurants.

- As you track you will identify high caloric or poor food selections.

- You may experience binge eating.

- Your scale may not move, but this is part of the process; your body composition may be changing.

- Identify if you eat when bored or stressed.

- You may be able to meet exercise requirements but struggle with nutrition.

- By the end of the third week you will have developed solutions to challenges.

Weeks 4 to 8

- You now are identifying poor food selection and making healthy choices.

- Fewer binges with trigger foods.

- Finding healthful alternatives to eating when bored or stressed.

- You will experience one or two weeks of weight fluctuation as you are still learning how to stay under your weekly caloric budget.

- You are finding the best exercises to meet your schedule and hitting expenditure goals.

- Staying under your caloric budget is still challenging but improving.

- You recognize trends in your weekly tracker that need improvement.

- Weight loss is trending down.

Weeks 9 to 12

- Traveling or life events may occur that cause you to "break even."

- You start weekly food prep.

- You start exploring other equipment or exercises that hit calories.

- Certain foods become boring, prompting you to explore other foods.

- Due to weight loss, you need to buy new clothes.

- Weight is still trending down.

Reminders and tips:

You want to reach your long-term weight with your short-term benchmarks.

Every 12 weeks, you can review your successes and challenges.

It's important to note: Not everyone will be able to hit one pound of weight loss per week in the beginning.

It's 110% possible to hit your goal with a half pound weight loss per week; the key is consistency.

Always looks for trends in areas where the Bodyscuplter's tracker shows you need improvement.

For example, it may be committing to an extra workout versus trying to make up for a caloric deficit in your nutrition.

It can also be noticing the weekends are most challenging so you decide to become more vigilant and create a meal plan for these days.

Also, for weeks that you are struggling with nutrition, remember that all is not lost!

You still have the metabolic effects from resistance training, meaning your body's ability to burn fat will increase at rest as long as you continue to have workouts that have progressive overloads. To maximize your hard work, you need to focus on your nutrition so you do not "break even."

If your weekly goal is missed, then you can review the trends and re-double your efforts.

Be sure to recognize small victories from your weekly Bodyscuplting Tracker:

- You progressed from thinking of beginning the program to actually tracking.

- You are doing better with trigger foods.

- You completed a workout and did not stop halfway through.

- You hit your daily goal for exercise, cardio, or nutrition either separately or together!

- You hit your weekly caloric deficit goal,

- Clothes are feeling big.

- You are "training smarter."

Maggie, Age 38, Female, Ht 5' 9", Sedentary Job, Full-Time Professional, Vegetarian.

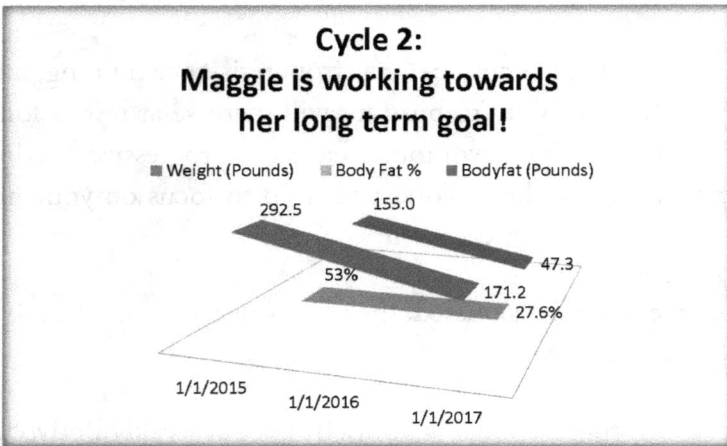

Cycle 2:
Maggie is working towards her long term goal!

■ Weight (Pounds) ■ Body Fat % ■ Bodyfat (Pounds)

292.5   155.0
53%   47.3
171.2
27.6%

1/1/2015   1/1/2016   1/1/2017

Example of Cycle 2

Start date 4/7/2015 at 292.5 pounds and 2 years later at 171.1 pounds, Maggie uses the A.I.M. Method to continue to body sculpt.

山

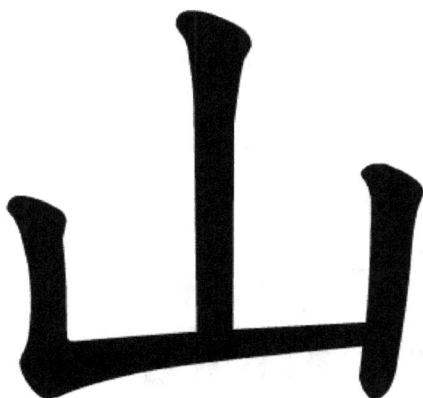

"The shortest way to do many things is to do only one thing at once."
– RICHARD CECIL

Chapter 11

THINGS TO REMEMBER AND THE SECRET TO LONG-TERM RESULTS

Making short-term weight loss goals along with a flexible and personalized program based on your body type and lifestyle = long-term results!

Things to remember after hitting your long-term goal (applies to short-term goals, too):

Be aware of your sugar intake (high glycemic foods) and make note of any continuous increase in cravings.

Be mindful of not drinking your calories! Some beverages are loaded with sugars and extra calories.

At this stage, choose healthful alternatives to sugary drinks and foods. Return to moderation and portion control.

Remember your TDEE especially after hitting your goals. Try not have three days in a row of going over by 500–1000 calories. Remember, one pound of fat is approximately 3,500 calories.

It takes about 21 days of inactivity from workouts to affect your metabolism and any lean muscle gains will have begun the process of atrophy.

I recommend going no more than 14 days between your workouts. Usually the initial motivation fades and old behaviors begin to return after 21 days, which makes it more difficult to return to the lifestyle that brought you the results.

The good news is that you have the tools and can jumpstart your program even after a long period of inactivity.

At this point, reassess and return to activities that are conducive to your TDEE If you are five pounds over then prevent additional weight gain.

You have now learned how to "BREAK OUT of breaking even"! Similar to what happens with a good book, each time you return to it you may learn or pick up on something new.

Experience is a great teacher; what you comprehend from the first time you read this book you may understand more after a few weeks of practicing the **A.I.M. Method.**

I would like to stress that it's normal to feel your goals are insurmountable, but the reality is your actions will lead to your results.

So practice the **A.I.M. Method**—especially on days you feel discouraged or not motivated!

You may be surprised how your feeling of wellness improves after taking action.

Lastly, I am going to share with you how you can truly maintain long-term results.

Start the journey with another person or even a group.

After YOU hit your goals, share this book and support the journeys of others.

This is the secret that is universal and it is an absolute:

Helping another person will help you on many levels, reminding you of how uncomfortable it was in the beginning, and how it got better with time and practice.

You are living proof that change is possible and have the personal experience and tools to help others achieve their goals.

Thank you for participating in the "BREAK OUT of breaking even" program.

Be well and Stay ACTIVE!

Julio A. Salado, NSCA C.P.T
TRX & Kettlebell Instructor.
USAW & USAPL Coach
Fitness Foundry designed for healthy living©.
Founder, Assess, Initiate, Motivate
email: juliosalado@fitnessfoundry.net

Simplify your "BREAK OUT of breaking even" program.
Get one to one support, save time and
keep the weight off!

If you are waiting for the perfect time to get started,
the time is now.

Sign up, it's free* www.fitnessfoundry.net

*Enter code BOBE2017

山

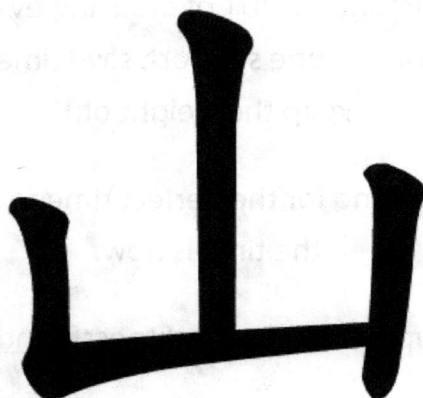

"We cannot teach people anything.
We can only help them discover it
within themselves."
— GALILEO GALILEI

Chapter 12

ABOUT THE AUTHOR

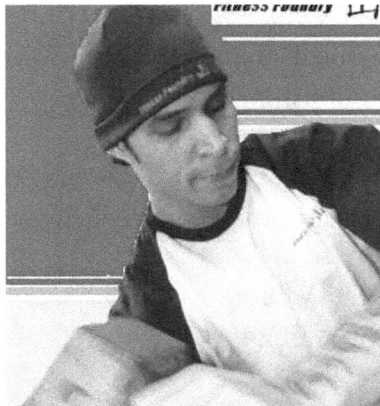

Specialties:

Julio Salado—National Strength & Conditioning Assoc.—
Certified Personal Trainer., U.S.A.W. Olympic Lifting Coach,
U.S.A.P.L. Powerlifting Coach, TRX & Kettle bell Certified
Instructor, National Assoc. of Sports Medicine Corrective Exercise Specialist, Certified Pre-Post Natal & Tai Chi Chuan 22
Form Instructor.

Training Philosophy:

My personal training is based on exercise science and holistic arts. I am also a mentor, educator and continuing education provider.

My experience is over 10 years of experience in cross-training with disciplines in bodybuilding, Olympic lifts, post-rehab training, senior fitness, sports performance & Tai Chi Chuan. I have successfully worked with clients 18-92 years of age from different backgrounds, pre-conditions, fitness levels and goals.

My health & fitness essays and videos have been published in print and online such as "Boston Mayor Marty Walsh's Senior Count TV Show," Boston.com 'Health and Family Magazine,' "Fitness Professional Online," "Boston Globe," "Boston Magazine" and "Top Personal Trainers Answer Your Questions" published by Regency Publishing.

No one is exempt from the benefits of living their dreams. Witness the results and experience the benefits of investing in yourself.

Be well and stay ACTIVE!!
Julio A. Salado, NSCA C.P.T
USAW & USAPL Coach
Fitness Foundry designed for healthy living©.
Founder
Assess, **I**nitiate, **M**otivate
www.fitnessfoundry.net

As seen on...

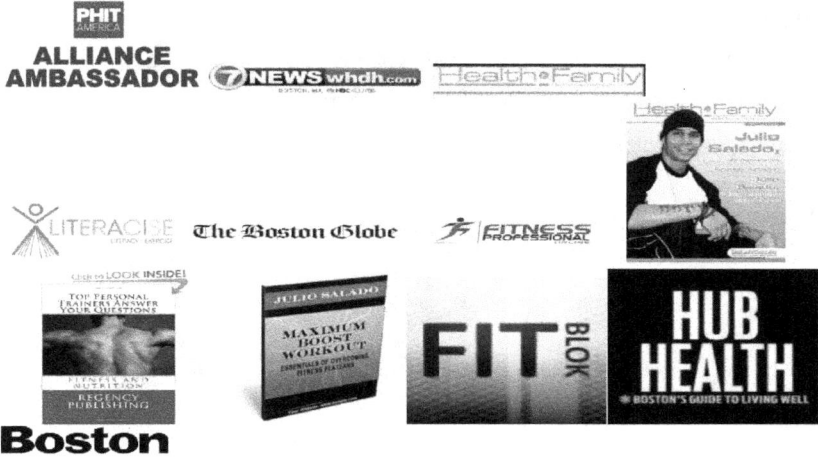

Testimonials:

"Training with Julio Salado has had nothing but positive effects for me. In my sport/profession you need to have strength, endurance, and be able to prevent injury. Using the unique exercises Julio has created, I have been able to reach a level of competition I never imagined was possible. I recommend Julio to anyone who is serious about their health and looking to take their life to the next level..." Matt G. Founder of Rhythm Snowboards

"Julio Salado is a talented trainer who helped me, even when I thought I could not be helped. I have always worked out in a variety of classes and activities. Julio's training really focused me on exercises to work out smarter, that is, to focus on my own strengths and weaknesses. His easy-going manner and extensive knowledge have helped me attain surprising results: weight loss (without really trying), overall strengthening and an improvement in motor function, despite some serious medical issues. What more could you ask from a trainer? " Jean C. PhD., RN.

山

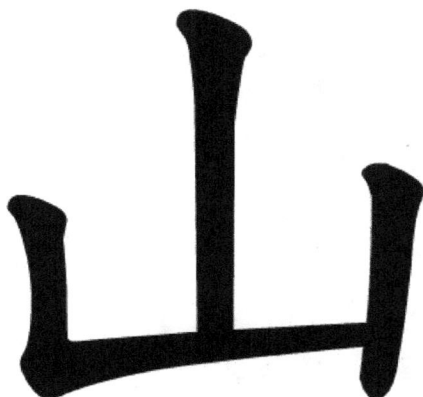

"Stronger Together!"

Chapter 13

FORMULAS, BODYSCULPTING REFERENCE SHEET, TRACKER, WORKOUT SHEET

Use this equation if you know your body fat percentage.

I prefer to use the "Katch-McArdle equation" because it utilizes your Lean Body Mass (LBM):

We first need to find out your lean muscle mass.

For easy reference, let's use Candie's answers:

- Age 35, Ht 5' 6" or 167.6 cm* Current Weight 200 Pounds or 90 Kilos, Body Fat 30%

- *Use this formula (Height inches x 2.54) to convert your height to centimeters.*

- Exercises 1 to 2 times per week, sedentary lifestyle

- Short-term weight loss goal: 190 pounds

- Long-term weight loss goal: 180 pounds

Body fat in pounds equation: Weight x BF%= body fat pounds. Example: 200 x .3 = 60.6 pounds of body fat

Lean Body Mass (LBM) equation: Weight – BF = LBM Example: 200 pounds – 60.6 pounds = 139.4 pounds LBM

"Katch-McArdle BMR equation" using Lean Body Mass (LBM):

370 + (21.6 x lean body mass in kilograms) = BMR in calories

To convert pounds to kilograms = (LBM) x .45 =kg. Example: 139.4 x .45= 62.7 kg LBM

Using Candie's data with the Katch McArdle equation:

370 + (21.6 x 62.7kg) = 1724 calories (BMR)

Please insert your data from the questionnaire into the Katch-McArdle equation":

Exercise D2

Current weight in pounds:	Current weight in kilograms:
370 + (21.6 x kg) =	
Your Basal Metabolic Rate =	

Once we establish your BMR we can then compare the rate to how many calories you are consuming versus the necessary caloric intake that's conducive to your weight loss goal.

Now let's learn how many calories you need to **MAINTAIN** your **CURRENT** weight. This is also known as your **TDEE** or Total Daily Energy Expenditure.

Simply multiply your BMR above by this standard Physical Activity Level (**PAL**):

- 1.2 = you are sedentary and do little or no exercise

- 1.375 = you exercise lightly or do sport 1–3 days/week

- 1.55 = you are moderately active and do exercise or a sport 3–5 days/week

- 1.725 = you are very active with hard exercise or a sport 6–7 days a week

- 1.9 = you are extremely active with very hard exercise or sport and a physical job or training twice a day

- The general population is at the 1.2 or 1.375 level.

We can use Candie's answers as an example:

- Candie's BMR is 1,724 calories and she exercises 1 to 2 times per week, sedentary lifestyle

- Candie's physical activity level (PAL) = 1.375 (exercise lightly or do a sport 1–3 days/week)

- Candie's Total Daily Energy Expenditure (TDEE) = 1,724 x 1.375 = **2,370 calories TDEE**

If Candie does NOT want to lose weight then she can continue to consume up to 2,370 calories daily.

Let's find out your TDEE:

Exercise F2

Your BMR=	Your PAL =
BMR x PAL = TDEE	
_____ x _____ =	Your TDEE =

Online calculator at www.fitnessfoundry.net

STOP! Using the above data, please go to page 108, Bodysculpting Reference Sheet and complete "Part A."

BODYSCULPTING REFERENCE SHEET

By Julio Salado
NSCA-CPT, USAW, USAPL

Name:

Part A:	Part A:
Baseline Data:	Short Term Goal:
Date:	New Weight:
Initial Weight:	Goal Body Fat%: _____ %
Body Fat %: _____ %	Calories need to burn to reach goal:
BMR:	Timetable: _____ weeks losing
Lean Body Mass: ____ pounds	____ pound per week
	Long Term Goal:
	New Weight: ____ pounds
	Goal Body Fat%: _____ %
	Calories needed to burn to reach
	goal: _____
	Timetable: ___ weeks losing
	_____ pounds per week
Part B1:	Part C:
Nutrition Plan:	Weekly total caloric deficit from
(TDEE) Daily caloric intake	exercise:
to maintain INITIAL weight:	You want to meet or exceed these
	numbers for the week.
_____	
Part B2:	Cardio:
You want to stay at or below these	
number: _____	Workouts:
Total calories for the day:	
	Other:
_____	
Total of calories for the week:	
_____	
Part B3:	
Suggested Macros for Nutrition:	
Protein ___ %	
Carbohydrates ___ %	
Fats _____ %	

Online sheet available at www.fitnessfoundry.net

BODYSCULPTING TRACKER

By Julio Salado
NSCA-CPT, USAW, USAPL

Weekly totals: Add up caloric expenditure for seven days of exercise and caloric daily nutrition, weigh in, and identify successes and challenges.

	Initial	Week 1	Week 2	Week 3	Week 4	Week 5	Week 6
Date							
Weight							
Nutrition							
Cardio							
Workout							
Other							

	Week 7	Week 8	Week 9	Week 10	Week 11	Week 12	
Date							
Weight							
Nutrition							
Cardio							
Workout							
Other							

Estimated Pounds Per Week:

	Initial	Week 1	Week 2	Week 3	Week 4	Week 5	Week 6
Date							
Weight							
Nutrition							
Cardio							
Workout							
Other							

	Week 7	Week 8	Week 9	Week 10	Week 11	Week 12	
Date							
Weight							
Nutrition							
Cardio							
Workout							
Other							

Notes:

Name:		Sample "BREAKING OUT of breaking even" Workout Sheet					
Dynamic Warm Ups/ Stretches							
Day 1	Circuit Training 3–4 Exercises with set caloric expenditure	Date/ Weight/ /Calories Burned	Date/ Weight/ /Calories Burned	Date/ Weight/ /Calories Burned	Date/ Weight/ /Calories Burned	Date/ Weight/ /Calories Burned	Date/ Weight/ Calories Burned

Day 2	Cardio with set time and caloric expenditure 2–3 Selections	Date/Time Calories Burned	Date/Time/Calories Burned	Date/Time/Calories Burned	Date/Time/Calories Burned	Date/Time/Calories Burned	Date/Time/Calories Burned
Day 3	Circuit Training 3–4 Exercises with set caloric expenditure	Date/Weight//Calories Burned	Date/Weight//Calories Burned	Date/Weight//Calories Burned	Date/Weight//Calories Burned	Date/Weight//Calories Burned	Date/Weight//Calories Burned

Notes:

Chapter 14

SERVICES, SOCIAL MEDIA, CONTACT

Fitness Foundry Services:

- Online Weight Loss Programs

- 1:1 Personal Training

- Personal and Group Training

- Elite Training for Sports Professionals

- Post Rehabilitation Training

- Group instruction for Beginner's Yang Tai Chi Chuan

- Group workshops and events on health, fitness, and nutrition

- Consultation on Personal Training Business Management

- Continue Education Provider Workshops

Website: www.fitnessfoundry.net

Website: www.breakoutofbreakingeven.com

Facebook: www.facebook.com/fitnessfoundry

Also www.facebook.com/breakoutofbreakingeven

Twitter: www.twitter.com/fitnessfoundry

Instagram: www.instagram.com/fitnessfoundryUSA

Email: juliosalado@fitnessfoundry.net

Simplify your "BREAK OUT of breaking even" program. Get one-to-one support, save time, and keep the weight off!

If you are waiting for the perfect time to get started, the time is now.

Sign up, it's free* www.fitnessfoundry.net

*Enter code BOBE2017